I0441087

Budget

Calories

Buy your food with Calories

for your health sake,

And to restore your true

body image!

Dr Marius *Potgieter*

Foreword

Some time ago I woke up to the realisation that, if you are overweight, there are not many things in life more important for you to do than to make every effort to lose weight, and a great gift you can offer to those you care for is to help them to do so too. I started to give this priority in our family, and the reason I wrote this book is because I saw that the application of the guidelines contained in it really work. Please consider giving it absolute priority for you and your family too!

There are of course other ways to go about it, but I can assure you from personal experience that if you diligently follow the method described in BUDGET CALORIES it will work for you, even if other methods have failed you. It is a self-help book for those who like to take an active part in 'navigation', and for those who do not like to be 'spoon fed' all the time, as many well-tried programs do. The first thing you have to do, however, is to decide to make losing weight an absolute priority for you and those you care for. Then you will find out how much better it is to eat to live in stead of living to eat. This book will not tell you all the reasons why you need to lose weight – you know them already – but it will describe a unique method of doing so.

To those who really want to lose weight but just cannot stick to a healthy diet, you need to find something to do that makes you excited, inspires you, and helps you not to depend on eating for comfort. Hold on to a picture in your mind of your ideal or 'core' body shape, and know this is the 'real' you, not the one you may see in the mirror at present. Your true image need not be model-perfect; just you as you ought to look.

Though Budget Calories is full of healthy suggestions; it does not give formal advice on health issues or, for that matter, on a specific diet. It is a method for implementing any diet you may choose.

This is the idea: your 'core' daily amount of necessary calories is equated to your income. If you spend more than your income, you have to do it with borrowed money, which puts you into debt. In our equation, this is represented by weight added to your ideal or core weight, which you have to carry around.

If you 'purchase' the food you eat daily strictly within your calorie allowance, I feel confident that you will 'get out of debt' from 'overspending' your calories reflected in excess weight. By sticking to your budget – that is, your 'core food intake' – you will reach or keep your 'core' or ideal weight.

Apart from sticking to your budget, try to enjoy your five-a-day fruit and vegetables. Get the nicest fruits and prepare your vegetables as attractively as possible. Eat enough roughage, be careful with your saturated fat and salt intake, and drink lots of water or nonsugary fluids, replacing the artificial with natural fresh food and juice.

Spread your meals by budgeting for low-calorie snacks in between. Earn 'extra income' with healthy exercise for 'spending' or 'saving'. **Spending** in this sense means buying items outside your budget (see later) and **saving** would be not spending what you earn by exercising, but keeping it and, by that, 'paying off some of your debt' (excess weight) quicker. Exercise as much as possible, and with as many of your muscles as possible, in order to lose fat and not muscle.

Earn 'extra

income' with

healthy exercise

for 'spending' or

'saving'

If you are part of a family, try to see the program as a 'family business'.

Although you will find it difficult to apply the specific measures you use to others at the same time, they will benefit from what you do. If you are in charge, you will be better informed when you prepare and dish up food. The rest of the family will be more inclined to follow your guidance as they see you getting into shape. It is very difficult to enforce a weight-loss diet on one member of a family. It will make it easier if the others eat according to their ideal core food amount as well.

I do not want anyone to go on a 'guilt trip' about their weight, or become obsessed by their diet. It should rather be seen as coming back to the normal, rather than implementing something abnormal. Eating too much is abnormal, as is spending outside your budget. None of us is perfect and though this should not be offered as an excuse for not sticking to our budget, it should help us not to feel too guilty when there are times when we don't. Just keep your mind on your real or 'core' image.

Kilojoules x 0.24 =

k/calories indicated by the

word calories and 'pay' relate

to paying with calories

Inches/cm converter

http://manuelsweb.com/ft_in_cm.htm

lb/kg tables

http://www.occupationalhealth.co

Before you can start, you have to have a clear idea of where you are weight- wise and where you want to be.

Find a BMI Calculator on Google (Medscape)

Make a note of this and, at the link below, have a look at your present and ideal body shapes if you want to
http://www.healthyweightforum.org/eng/calculators/bmi-visual-graph/

How to Budget for Your Food Intake with Calories

The idea of budgeting with calories is simple but unique.

Because it is simple, it is easy to follow.

Because it is unique, people who have tried and failed at other ways to lose or maintain weight have not tried this one!

This is not so much about losing weight as it is on how to budget with your amount of **core calories** to 'purchase' your healthy or **core weight**. If you realise this, you do not have to get on the scales regularly – just at the beginning and then occasionally to see if you are still on track.

Do you want to give it a go? First, let me tell you how I came upon the idea.

Travelling on holiday with our family, we decided to give everyone a certain amount of money for food in the morning; they could do whatever they wanted with it. It was actually a lot of fun to see how saving money for dinner influenced everyone's choices of lunch and snacks during the day! Without this plan, our expenditure on food would not have been under control, resulting in more spending on our bodies (money and weight-wise).

Traditional dieting revolves around saving on calories; this one is about spending them according to your budget. Let us assume that the basic calorie requirement for an adult is more or less 10 calories per pound per day for a woman and 12 calories per pound per day for a man, not taking the level of activity and exercising into account. That is the basic number of calories you have to consume to prevent your body from going into a 'hunger mode'.

To begin with, take your **present weight** in pounds, e.g. 180 lbs. of body weight.

For a woman allow 180 x 10 = 1800 calories per day.

For a man allow 180 x 12 = 2160 calories per day.

This is your **starting budget** and for obtaining your core weight ASAP we are not going to consider your normal activity level for now. In other words, this will be the amount of calories needed to support your present weight even if you are inactive.

You have already looked, a few pages back, at what your 'normal' or 'core' weight should be to come into your normal BMI range. For instance, if you are a woman and your ideal or core weight is 130 lbs, slowly come down to 130 x 10 = 1300 calories. If you are not losing enough for your liking, come down to 1200 per day (never less than 1100) for a while and keep at it until you reach your core weight. Then continue 'spending' only your core calories to keep your core weight stable, but from then on, add calories according to your level of activity.

If you come down from 1800 calories to 1300 calories, you won't 'feed' 50lbs of your body's weight and you will gradually lose it.

For a man, to keep your **present weight,** for instance if you weigh 180lbs x 12 = 2160 calories, it will take 6 days to reach your core daily amount of calories when decreasing it by 100 calories per day, if your core weight is 130lbs x 12 = 1560 calories

Whenever you regularly spend calories 'above your income', you run into 'debt.' The idea is, therefore, that you try to spend only your core amount of calories to attain your core or ideal weight.

If you want to look again at what your core or ideal body shape might look like according to your BMI, go back to the link and keep your mind on your **ideal image**. A good idea is also to print out the BMI graphics and see how you come down 'figure by figure' until you get to where you want to be.

This leads us to an **alternative method,** which is what I call the 'stepping down' method that you can use if you find you are getting too hungry when getting straight down to the core calories, especially if there is a big difference between your initial and ideal core weight.

When you look at the graphic BMI, which you should have printed and ideally pasted on your fridge, you will notice that if you are a woman and your height is 5 feet 2 inches, a BMI of 24, which is within normal range, gives you a core weight of 130lbs. A BMI of 22, which gives you a core weight of 120lbs x 10 = 1200, will be your lowest calorie intake, so as not to go into 'hunger mode.' This you will use if you want to lose weight as fast as possible.

If, as we have previously discussed your initial weight may be 180lbs (180 x 10 = 1800 calories: BMI 33) you may prefer to use the 'step down method' than to go to 1300 cal per day in a week or so. Aim for stepping down one image at a time, e.g. from a BMI of 33 to 29, by buying your food with the calories of the second image down – that is the BMI of 26 or 140 x 10 = 1400 calories per day. (You can still decrease your daily calories by 100 and it will take 4 days) As soon as you reach the BMI and image of 29, you aim for 26 by using the calories for the BMI of 24 and then for 22 to get to 24, which is your goal.

If you find even this method difficult, just go for the calories of the first BMI image below the one you are on. As soon as you reach the weight of that one, go to the next one down until you reach your goal. This will make you lose weight more slowly, but you should still lose it, as we are not taking your levels of activity into account. Except of course those that you do for extra 'income.'

In summary then, there are three ways to get from the amount of calories that keep your initial weight going to that which you need for your ideal core weight

- I suggest that to be a weight for a BMI of 24.

1. The fastest way is going down from your initial weight calories by 100 calories per day, until you reach the number of daily calories for your core weight.

2. The moderate way is taking the BMI graphic images and aim for the one just below where you are, but calculate the daily calories for the BMI of two images down.

3. The slow way is to aim for and calculate your calories for the BMI

of the image just below the one where you are.

You may choose any of the methods and may even 'mix and match'. The idea is that you should experience being in control of your weight-loss and maintenance program. In case you are someone whose weight is below normal, you can do it just the other way around, but again make sure that there is no medical or serious psychological reason for you being underweight; addressing this should take priority.

Multiplying the weight in lbs by 10 for women and 12 for men may not give the exact daily calorie requirement, but it is near enough and is a valuable working formula.

There may be variations in your daily food intake, but try to stick to an average; if you spend a bit more today, try to cut it down tomorrow. At least try to make your week balance; take for instance 1200 x 7 = 8400 calories per week.

Much of this you will have worked out for yourself.

As already mentioned, if you earn more calories with exercise, you can spend them to enjoy 'privileges' outside your budget or you can 'save' them in order to lose weight faster. Find articles in books and on the Internet that will teach you the best way to walk and do other exercises.

Start with the number

of calories to feed your

present weight and

decrease them steadily to

feed only your ideal or

core weight

The second important aspect is not only to keep to your ideal core calorie spending, but also to 'spend' the calories selectively. Of course, you have to spend your calories on a healthy balanced diet, but you also need to eat in a way that enables you to keep your insulin levels as stable as possible, by introducing carbohydrates with a low glycemic index, considering the glycemic load also, to replace those with a high glycemic index. (An excellent book on this with recipes is, "Glycemic Index Cookbook" from Publications International Ltd)

The reason for keeping your insulin levels stable is that a too high or a too low level of insulin can affect your metabolism and cause your body to store more fat, especially internal fat (in and around your organs), which may be increased even if you look slim from the outside and which may affect your health.

Also by better spacing of your meals and snacks throughout the day you will keep your insulin level more stable.

If you are **exercising moderately**, you can add 300 calories to your core daily amount. Ideally, after you have reached your core weight – we don't want you to become skinny!

If you think you will not be able to stick to this by yourself, put someone else in control of the cookies! Alternatively, get others to work with you.

Even when you follow this plan, you must still remember to stick to a balanced food intake, which is broadly:

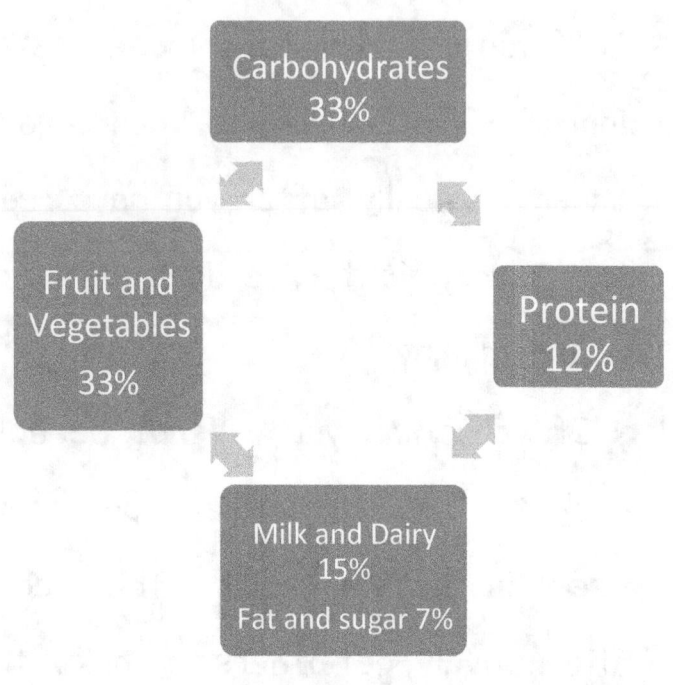

Keep this in mind when you follow your daily budget.

Let us look at it as follows:

Of 1200 calories:

144   Protein (excluding the protein in milk and dairy products);

396 Carbohydrates;

396 Fruits and Vegetables;

180 Milk and Dairy;

84 Fats and Sugars.

Of course, you don't have to be rigid as far as the categories are concerned but keep them in mind when you make your choices of food during the day and throughout the week. Take special care not to miss your five a day fruit and vegetables; the others usually look after themselves.   However, you still have to stick to your core amount of calories per day.

Make a list of the calories in the food you use daily until you remember them.

Approximate values of a few are:

Full cream milk in coffee or tea = 25 cal, teaspoon sugar = 20 cal, margarine on bread = 27cal, jam = 25 cal, apple = 80 cal, juice – best to look on the box or bottle, egg, depending on size = 90 cal.

If you have breakfast with oats and a piece of toast, it may add up like this: 40gm oats = 150 cal, the half-cream milk added to prepare it = 50 cal, margarine on it = 27 cal, sugar if you want to = 20 cal (247) toast = 60 cal, margarine (Bertolli) = 27 cal, cheese spread = 25 cal, marmalade = 25 cal (137), total = 384 cal spent on your breakfast and a cup of coffee with milk and one teaspoon sugar will cost you another 45 cal = 429 cal.

You may decide if you want to spend all this on breakfast or rather leave out some of the items and have more to spend later. Also, for instance just a boiled egg with toast: toast = 60 cal, margarine = 27 cal, egg = 90 cal, total = 177 cal.

It is not a bad idea to budget for about 400 cal for breakfast, 300 cal for lunch and 600 cal for the evening meal if your daily budget is 1300 calories. To save for snacks in-between you can spend less on any of your main meals.

You will come a long way by looking at the packages and by using your scales if you have a set. For further information, use any of the many websites. I think the best website to visit for getting your calorie values is:

http://www.caloriecounting.co.uk/resourc es/intro.htm

If you wish, especially during the time that you are trying to lose weight, you can use some of the carbohydrate calories for a bit more protein. For instance, depending on the size, you will have to 'spend' your whole protein allowance on a single chicken fillet. Maybe you would like two, or another piece of meat or fish?

Keep in mind that a full English breakfast may set you back about 560 calories. If you do have one now and then making you to overspend, you can earn some calories with exercise or subtract the over spent amount from the daily allowance for the next 7 days, e.g. 50 calories less per day will make up for 350 calories. Fortunately for you, if you are a man you have more calories to spend e.g. 130lb x 12 = 1560, which is 260 calories more than for a woman with the same weight (130 x 10 = 1300 calories) so it will make it easier to 'pay' for the breakfast - just be careful of the fat and sugar however.

It is important to check on the sugar content of the carbohydrates you eat (5gm/100gm is low and 15gm per 100gm is high.) Try to stay between these values and, for an adult, take no more than 90g sugar per day, bearing in mind that many non-sugary foods contain some sugar anyhow.

Sugar may, of course, affect your teeth as well and, in this regard, it is better to eat whole fruit rather than drinking juice.

During the day you can do certain 'tasks' to 'supplement your budget'. These will be the physical activities you are involved in. Treat yourself with these outside of your core budget. For example, if you weigh 170 lbs (just over 12 stone) and you walk at 4 miles per hour you can have a 330ml can of Coke, if you need one now and then, after 21 minutes of walking (139 calories). Walking for 30 minutes gives you 198 calories extra to spend or save: if you overspent on your budget, you will have to do some 'moonlighting!'

Don't you think this can be fun?

The Internet is full of information about how to calculate the amount of calories you can earn extra with different activities.

When your core calorie intake is right, you will in time reach your core weight; then you won't have to get on the scales all the time, you can just get on with your life. In the same way, that happiness is a by-product of engaging in something that results in it, you cannot pursue happiness itself.

The fact is also that each person is an individual with a metabolism that may be different for one reason or another. If after a few weeks, you find that your weight does not drop, even when you have stopped 'feeding' your excess weight, your core amount of calories may be lower than your estimation. Decrease them by another 100 calories per day and weigh yourself weekly for a while.

Only make further adjustments if, on two consecutive weeks, you have gained or failed to lose some weight. You may then decrease your daily calorie expenditure by another 100 calories (but never below 1100-1200, depending on your size) or increase your exercise if possible.

While you learn how to adjust your lifestyle, you will have to make calculations regularly, but later as you get to know your values, it will become easier.

Become so calorie and

health literate that the

selection of the right

food will be as natural a

part of your life as

breathing.

Four helpful devices that you may want to invest in are:

1. A set of calorie scales such as the Nutriscales from Lloyd's pharmacy, also available from Amazon. (You will anyhow need to have a set of kitchen scales to be able to weigh your food). With the Nutriscales you can see, for instance, that there are 107 calories in a large egg weighing 71 grams, as well as 9.2 grams of protein, 0.6 grams of carbohydrate, and 7.2 grams of fat, 2.3 of which is saturated. A little booklet is provided giving codes for

each food item. It is a bit of a pain to look them up and punch them in, but it does help. Fortunately, on most food packaging, you will find the amount of calories etc, but you will still need the scales.

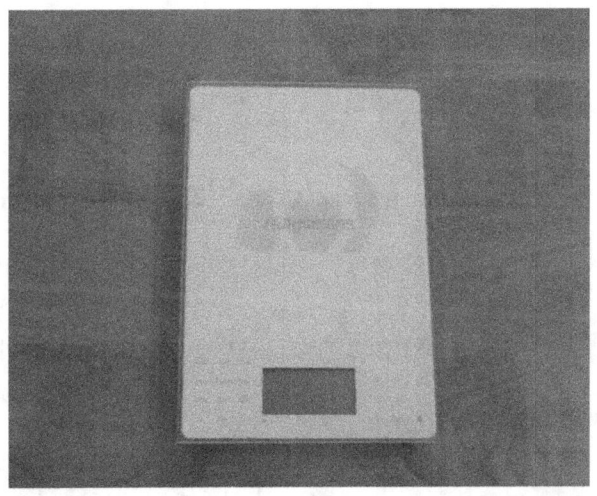

2. A calculator is the most useful tool. You may use your mobile phone or

whatever. I found a calculator that gives a print-out, which is very handy, the Aurora PR710 from Amazon. It prints in two colours for + and -. Start the day with, for instance, 1200 + and key in a negative value every time you buy something to eat. You will clearly see how many calories you still have available to spend and you will be able to have a print out of your 'bill'.

I recommend you keep this calculator in the kitchen rather than on the dining-room table if you are not alone; others may not appreciate you 'preparing your bill' at the table! You can do this in the kitchen, before or after the meal.

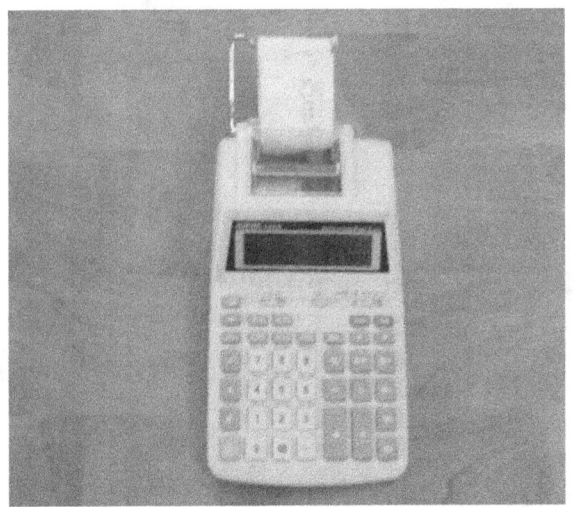

3. A pedometer will help you to know how many calorie points you gain during normal and specific activities.

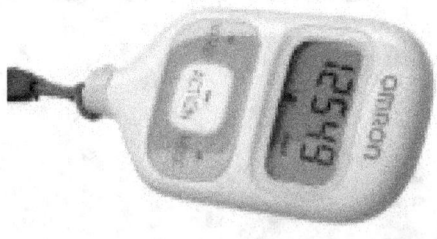

4. A journal, in which you write down the important an interesting points about your challenge to get back and keep your 'birth-right' shape!

Kitchen set-up with

calculator and scales ready

for action.

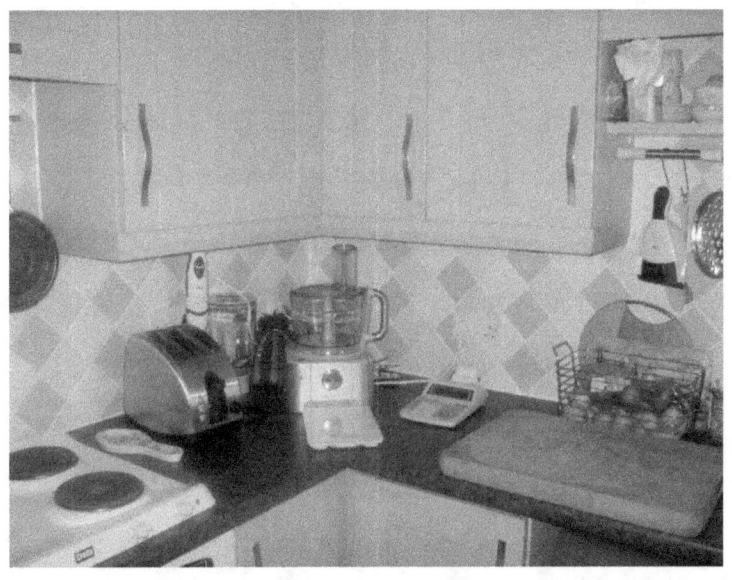

SIX STEPS TO BETTER HEALTH

AND BODY HAPPINESS

1. START TODAY BY BUYING FOOD WITH YOUR CALORIE ALLOWANCE (CORE AMOUNT OF CALORIES FOR YOUR PRESENT WEIGHT). MAKE SURE TO EAT APPROPRIATE PORTIONS OF YOUR 5 FRUITS AND VEGETABLES PER DAY AND, AS FAR AS POSSIBLE, EAT FOODS WITH A LOW GI RATHER THAN THOSE WITH A HIGH GI. SPREAD YOUR MEALS OVER THE DAY BY ADDING SNACKS BETWEEN MEALS AND AT BED TIME. EAT ENOUGH ROUGHAGE.

2. AFTER YOU HAVE MANAGED TO STAY WITHIN YOUR CALORIE ALLOWANCE FOR MAINTAINING YOUR PRESENT WEIGHT, MOVE SLOWLY TO YOUR IDEAL CORE AMOUNT OF CALORIES PER DAY. AS ALREADY MENTIONED YOU MAY DECREASE YOUR SPENDING ALLOWANCE BY 100 CALORIES PER

DAY. ADJUST YOUR SPENDING ON YOUR PRESENT WEIGHT, FOR EACH MEAL OR SNACK, DO THAT FOR YOUR IDEAL CORE WEIGHT. DON'T BE IN A HURRY, BUT DON'T CONTINUE WASTING YOUR CALORIES (AND MONEY) ON THE EXTRA WEIGHT YOU HAVE TO CARRY AROUND.

3. DRINK LOTS OF WATER OR LOW-SUGAR DRINKS.

4. YOU NEED ONLY TO WEIGH YOURSELF ONCE A MONTH WHEN YOU ARE SURE YOU ARE BUYING AND EATING YOUR CORE DIET.

5. IF YOU CANNOT RESIST BUYING CERTAIN FOODS AND OVERSPEND, GET SOMEONE TO RATION YOU, OR EARN EXTRA CALORIES WITH EXERCISE ASAP. IF YOU REALLY CANNOT STICK TO THE PROGRAM, GET SOMEONE TO HELP, AS WITH A 'DEBT MANAGEMENT PLAN'.

6. IF YOU ARE HEALTHY, YOU SHOULD EAT BECAUSE YOU ARE HUNGRY. DON'T WASTE FOOD BY PUTING TOO MUCH ON YOUR PLATE, BUT NEVER FEEL OBLIGATED TO FINISH EVERYTHING ON YOUR PLATE WHEN YOU ARE NO LONGER HUNGRY. DO NOT, HOWEVER, MAKE A HABIT OF LEAVING CERTAIN FOODS, BECAUSE THEN YOUR DIET WILL BECOME UNBALANCED. DISPOSE OF UNWANTED FOOD AS IT MAY ONLY GATHER 'DEBT' AS IT GOES THROUGH YOU, AND THEN GETS DISPOSED OF ANYWAY. ON THE OTHER HAND BE HAPPY IF YOU ARE BIT HUNGRY AFTER A MEAL!

If we think about it, to be subjected to the detrimental effect of eating more than our core amount of food is not worthwhile. Our chances of developing heart disease, hypertension, stroke, diabetes, cancer and Alzheimer's, are higher when we are overweight. Also, why pay for carrying with us an unnecessary burden?

Have a look at the economics:

http://www.mymoneyblog.com/whatdoes-200-Calories-cost-theeconomics-of-obesity.html

It makes economic sense to eat to support your core weight instead of your excess weight. Spending money on expensive programs on how to lose weight is like paying twice for your food!

To keep 50 lbs of excess
weight going will costs you
about £10 per week, that
means you spend about £520
per year for carrying around
an unnecessary burden

Have fun and please send me your comments at bestcanbe@googlemail.com

If you want to have a look at my other books, you will find them on Amazon under my name

Afterword

I have written this book as a popular workbook, and though I have taken precautions to convey correct information, I do not make any claim for it to be a medical textbook.

To conclude, I would like to emphasise three important points:

1. If you have a health problem, talk to your GP before embarking on this program.
2. This book is written primarily for adults who are able to take responsibility for themselves.
3. Staying within the accepted BMI (Body Mass Index) range is still the 'gold standard', but remember the possibility of 'internal fat.' and that you may adjust upwards for muscle volume.

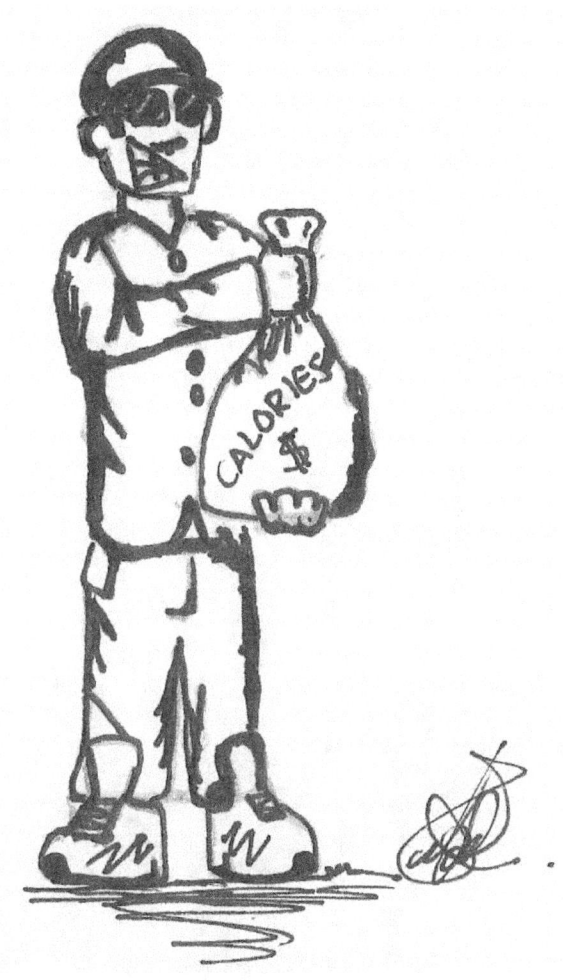

Good luck!

www.ingramcontent.com/pod-product-compliance
Lightning Source LLC
Chambersburg PA
CBHW071244280526
45788CB00004B/1576